# Secrets beyond Chair Yoga for Weight Loss

The benefits of weight loss for stroke prevention

Dr. Martin XAvier

Copyright © 2022 CP Print All rights reserved

The characters and events portrayed in this book are fictitious. Any similarity to real persons, living or dead is coincidental and not intended by the author.

No part of this book may be reproduced, or stored in a retrieval system, or transmitted in any form or by any means, electronic, mechanical, photocopying, recording, or otherwise, without express written permission of the publisher.

ISBN: 9798325845765
Imprint: Independently published

Cover design by: Art Painter Librar Congress Control Number: 2018675309

Printed in the United States of America

# DEDICATION

Dedicated to those on a journey towards better health and vitality. May this book serve as a guiding light, illuminating the path to weight loss and stroke prevention? With gratitude to the readers who embark on this voyage of self-discovery and empowerment.

For those seeking the transformative power of chair yoga, may this knowledge unlock the secrets to a healthier, happier life. Here's to embracing the wisdom and strength found beyond the poses, and discovering the boundless potential within.

May your dedication to wellness inspire others, and may your journey be filled with joy, peace, and abundant health.

# Table of Contents

**Weight Loss Strategies for Stroke Prevention** ..........................1

JAMES WILLIAM ..........................................................................1

DEDICATION ................................................................................3

INTRODUCTION. .........................................................................5

CHAPTER 1 ...................................................................................8

    The Mental and Emotional Benefits of Weight Loss. ............8

CHAPTER 2 .................................................................................12

    Benefits of Exante Products for Weight Loss......................12

CHAPTER 3 .................................................................................15

    The Benefits of Weight Loss . ................................................15

CHAPTER 4 .................................................................................18

    Successful campaigns to prevent laser skin cancer . ...........18

CHAPTER 5 .................................................................................22

    Predictive Models for Hearing Loss Prevention ..................22

CHAPTER 6 .................................................................................27

    Risk Factors for Hypertension and Stroke . .........................27

CHAPTER 7 .................................................................................30

    Risk Factors for Hypertension and Stroke. .........................30

CHAPTER 8 .................................................................................33

The link between high blood pressure and health risks. ........ 33
CHAPTER 9 .................................................................... 37
Medications for Hypertension and Stroke Prevention ............... 37
Lifestyle Changes to Control Hypertension and Prevent Stroke ...40
CHAPTER 11 .................................................................. 43
Genetic Links and Risk Reduction Strategies . ....................... 43
CHAPTER 12 .................................................................. 46
Signs and Symptoms of Hypertension . ............................... 46
CHAPTER 13 .................................................................. 49
Understanding Hypertension and its Link to Stroke ............ 49
CHAPTER 14 .................................................................. 53
Introduction to stroke and hypertension . ............................ 53
CHAPTER 15 .................................................................. 56
**The Risks of Stroke in Obese Individuals** ....................... 56
CHAPTER 16 .................................................................. 59
**Medications and Treatments for Blood Pressure Control** . ................................................................................... 59
CHAPTER 17 .................................................................. 65
Importance of Blood Pressure Management in Stroke Prevention . ................................................................... 65
CHAPTER 18 .................................................................. 68
Understanding Stroke and Its Risk Factors . ........................ 68
CHAPTER 19 .................................................................. 71
Blood pressure and cholesterol research . ........................... 71
CHAPTER 20 .................................................................. 74

Understanding the Connection . ............................................74
CHAPTER 21................................................................................77
Monitoring Blood Pressure and Stroke Risk . .......................77
CHAPTER 22................................................................................80
An overview ........................................................................80
CHAPTER 23................................................................................84
Types of Beta Blockers for Anxiety . ...................................84
CHAPTER 24................................................................................87
Mental Health Benefits and Emotional Renewal ................87
CHAPTER 25................................................................................90
A therapeutic hobby for body and mind . ..........................90

# INTRODUCTION.

Being overweight or obese is an important risk factor for stroke. According to the World Health Organization, obesity is a leading cause of preventable death worldwide. *The good news* is that losing just a few pounds can significantly reduce your risk of stroke. In this book, we will explore the benefits of weight loss for stroke prevention and some other best approaches towards effective weight loss campaign.

1. **Lower blood pressure**: *High blood pressure* is a major cause of stroke. Losing weight can help lower blood pressure, which reduces the risk of stroke. According to the American Heart *Association, losing just 5-10% of your body weight can significantly* lower blood pressure.

2. **Improved Cholesterol Levels**: High cholesterol levels can increase the risk of stroke. Losing weight can help improve cholesterol levels, reducing the risk of stroke. According to the *National Heart,* Lung, and Blood Institute, losing weight can

lower LDL (bad) cholesterol levels and increase HDL (*good*) *cholesterol levels*.

3. **Reduced risk of diabetes:** Obesity is a major risk factor for diabetes, which can increase the risk of stroke. Losing weight can help reduce the risk of diabetes, which reduces the risk of stroke. According to the *American Diabetes* Association, losing just 5-7% of your body weight can significantly reduce your risk of developing diabetes.

4. **Improved Heart *Health*:** Losing weight can improve heart health, reducing the risk of stroke. According to the American Heart Association, losing weight can reduce the risk of heart disease, which is a major risk factor for stroke.

5. ***Improved Mobility*:** Obesity can make it difficult to move, increasing the risk of falls and other accidents that can lead to a stroke. Losing weight can improve mobility, reducing the risk of falls and other accidents.

6. **Improved Mental Health:** Obesity can negatively impact mental health, increasing the risk of depression and anxiety. Losing weight can improve mental health and reduce the risk of stroke.

When it comes to weight loss for stroke prevention, there are several options to consider. One option is to make lifestyle changes, such as eating a healthy diet and exercising regularly. Another option is to join a weight-loss program, such as *Weight Watchers* or *Jenny Craig*. A third option is to consider weight loss surgery, such as gastric bypass or gastric sleeve.

While all of these options can be effective, lifestyle changes are often *the best option* for *long-term* weight loss and stroke prevention. They are durable and can be integrated into everyday life. Weight loss programs can be effective, but they can be expensive and may not be sustainable in *the long term*. Weight loss surgery can be effective, but it is invasive and carries risks.

Weight loss is an important step in preventing a stroke. Losing just a few pounds can significantly reduce the risk of stroke by improving blood pressure, cholesterol levels and heart health, reducing the risk of diabetes, improving mobility and improving mental health. When it comes to weight loss for stroke prevention, lifestyles changes are often *the best option not chair yoga*.

Chair yoga can be a valuable component of a weight loss journey but there are indeed several methods or approaches that are typically more effective for shedding pounds.

**Calorie Restriction:**

One of the most fundamental principles of weight loss is consuming fewer calories than you expend. This can be achieved by monitoring your calorie intake and making mindful choices about the foods you eat. For example, focusing on whole, nutrient-dense foods like fruits, vegetables, lean proteins, and whole grains can help you feel fuller on fewer calories compared to processed foods high in sugar and unhealthy fats.

**Regular Exercise:**

While chair yoga offers gentle movement and can improve flexibility and mobility, more vigorous forms of exercise tend to burn more calories and promote weight loss. Activities like brisk walking, jogging, cycling, swimming, and strength training can all contribute to burning calories and building lean muscle mass, which can increase your metabolic rate and support weight loss over time.

**High-Intensity Interval Training (HIIT):**

HIIT involves short bursts of intense exercise followed by brief periods of rest or lower-intensity activity. This type of workout has been shown to be particularly effective for burning calories and improving cardiovascular health. HIIT workouts can include exercises like sprinting, jumping jacks, burpees, or cycling at maximum effort for short intervals, making them a time-efficient option for weight loss.

**Mindful Eating:**

In addition to focusing on what you eat, paying attention to how you eat can also support weight loss. Practicing mindful eating involves slowing down, savoring each bite, and paying attention to your body's hunger and fullness cues. By eating more slowly and mindfully, you're more likely to recognize when you're satisfied and avoid overeating, which can contribute to weight loss.

**Behavioral Changes:**

Making sustainable lifestyle changes is essential for long-term weight loss success. This may involve setting realistic goals, creating a supportive environment, managing stress effectively, getting adequate sleep, and finding healthy ways to cope with emotions that don't involve food. Behavioral strategies like keeping a food journal, planning meals ahead of time, and seeking support from friends, family, or a healthcare professional can all enhance your weight loss efforts.

While chair yoga can be a valuable addition to a weight loss regimen, combining it with these more intensive methods may yield faster and more significant results. It's essential to choose approaches that align with your preferences, abilities, and lifestyle to create a sustainable plan for achieving your weight loss goals. So let's move into the full understanding of the benefits of weight loss for stroke prevention and all other illness.

# CHAPTER 1

## The Mental and Emotional Benefits of Weight Loss.

Losing weight is a journey that offers much more than just physical benefits. The mental and emotional benefits of weight loss can be just as important, if not greater, than the physical changes. From boosting self-esteem to improving mental health, weight loss can positively impact every aspect of a person's life. In this section we explore the many mental and emotional benefits of weight loss, and how they can contribute to a journey of personal growth.

**1. Improved self-esteem**

One of the most important mental benefits of weight loss is improved self-esteem. When a person loses weight, he or she often feels more confident in his appearance and abilities. This can lead to a more positive self-image, which can translate into better relationships, increased productivity and a more fulfilling life. For example, someone who previously felt too self-conscious to attend social gatherings may now feel more comfortable and confident in their appearance, leading to more meaningful connections with others.

## 2. Reduced stress and anxiety

Weight loss can also reduce stress and anxiety levels. Being overweight can cause stress on the body, which can lead to physical discomfort and emotional distress. Losing weight can alleviate these symptoms, leading to a more relaxed and peaceful state of mind. Additionally, exercise releases endorphins, which can improve mood and reduce stress levels. For example, someone who previously struggled with anxiety may find that regular exercise and a healthy diet help them manage their symptoms.

## 3. More energy and focus

Another mental benefit of weight loss is increased energy and focus. Losing weight often involves adopting healthier habits, such as regular exercise and a balanced diet. These habits can improve overall health and well-being, leading to higher energy levels and better focus. For example, someone who previously struggled with fatigue may find that they have more energy throughout the day, leading to higher productivity and a more satisfying life.

## 4. Improved mental health

Weight loss can also improve mental health. Studies have shown that losing weight can reduce symptoms of depression and anxiety and improve overall mental well-being. Additionally, adopting healthy habits can improve self-care, leading to better mental health outcomes. For example, someone who previously struggled with depression may find that regular exercise and a healthy diet help them manage their symptoms and improve their overall mental well-being.

5. **More self-confidence and motivation**

Finally, weight loss can increase self-confidence and motivation. When someone sets a weight loss goal and achieves it, he/she often feels a sense of achievement and pride. This can lead to increased self-confidence and motivation to continue making positive changes in their lives. Additionally, positive feedback and support from others can reinforce these feelings, leading to a more positive and fulfilling life. For example, a person who previously struggled with motivation may find that achieving their weight loss goal gives them the confidence and motivation to pursue other goals in their life.

The mental and emotional benefits of weight loss are numerous and can contribute to a journey of personal growth. From improved self-esteem to reduced stress and anxiety, weight loss can positively impact every aspect of a person's life. By adopting healthy habits and making positive changes, individuals can improve their mental and emotional well-being, leading to a more fulfilling and satisfying life.

# CHAPTER 2

**Benefits of Exante Products for Weight Loss.**
Exante Diet: How to Achieve Weight Loss Goals with Exante Products

Benefits of Exante Products for Weight Loss

Exante products are a great way to support weight loss goals and maintain a healthy lifestyle. These products are designed with the best ingredients to control hunger, increase metabolism and provide essential nutrients. In this blog section, we discuss the benefits of Exante weight loss products.

1. **Convenient and easy to use**

Exante products are convenient and easy to use, making them perfect for people with busy lives. They can be easily prepared in minutes and consumed on the go. This means you can stick to your weight loss goals even while you're on the go. Exante products come in a variety of forms, including shakes, bars, soups, and meals, making it easy to choose the one that suits your taste and preference.

2. **Low in calories and high in nutrients**

Exante products are low in calories and high in nutrients, making them perfect for people who want to lose weight. They are designed to provide all the essential nutrients the body needs while keeping calorie intake low. This means you can enjoy a balanced diet without having to worry about consuming too many calories. Exante products are also high in protein, which helps you feel full longer.

3. **Variety of flavors**

Exante products are available in different flavors, making it easy to find the one that suits your taste. They come in sweet and savory flavors, meaning you can enjoy your favorite foods while sticking to your weight loss goals. Some of the popular flavors include chocolate, vanilla, strawberry and banana.

4. **Adaptable plans**

Exante offers customizable plans tailored to your weight loss goals. You can choose from several plans, including total meal replacement, flexi and 5:2 intermittent fasting. Each plan is designed to **help you achieve your weight loss goals** while providing the necessary nutrients to keep you healthy.

5. **Affordable**

Exante products are affordable, making them accessible to anyone who wants to lose weight. They offer great value for money, especially when compared to other slimming products on the market. This means you can achieve your weight loss goals without spending a lot of money.

Exante products are a great way to support your weight loss goals. They are convenient, low in calories, high in nutrients, available in a variety of flavors and affordable. Customizable plans allow you to achieve your weight loss goals while enjoying a balanced diet.

# CHAPTER 3

### The Benefits of Weight Loss.

Losing weight can be a daunting task, but the benefits of weight loss are numerous. Not only does it improve physical health, but it also positively impacts mental health, self-esteem and overall quality of life. In this section we explore the many benefits of weight loss and how it can lead to a new lease on life.

1. **Improved physical health:** One of the most important benefits of weight loss is improved physical health. Losing weight can reduce the risk of developing chronic diseases such as diabetes, heart disease and stroke. It can also improve joint health and reduce the risk of developing arthritis. Additionally, weight loss can improve sleep quality, increase energy levels and reduce the risk of developing sleep apnea.

2. **Increased Self-Esteem:** Weight loss can also have a positive impact on mental health and self-esteem. Losing weight can increase self-confidence and self-esteem, leading to a more

positive outlook on life. It can also improve body image and reduce feelings of shame and embarrassment.

3. **Improved quality of life:** Weight loss can also lead to an overall improvement in quality of life. It can increase mobility and perform daily activities more easily. It can also improve social interactions and lead to a more active lifestyle, which can improve mental health and overall well-being.

4. **Better Mental Health:** Weight loss can also have a positive impact on mental health. It can reduce symptoms of depression and anxiety, improve mood and increase self-confidence. Additionally, weight loss can lead to a more positive body image, which can reduce feelings of shame and embarrassment.

5. **More energy:** Losing weight can also increase energy levels. With less weight to carry, the body requires less energy to perform daily activities, leading to greater endurance and endurance. This can lead to a more active lifestyle, which can improve overall health and well-being.

When it comes to weight loss, there are many options available. Some people choose to follow a strict diet and exercise regimen, while others opt for weight loss surgery. While both options can be effective, it is important to consider the risks and benefits of each option.

For those who choose to follow a diet and exercise regimen, it is important to consult with a healthcare provider to develop a safe and effective plan. This can be a combination of healthy eating habits, regular exercise and behavioral therapy.

For those opting for weight loss surgery, it is important to understand the risks and benefits. Although surgery can lead to significant weight loss, it also carries risks such as infection, bleeding, and complications during surgery. It is important to consult a healthcare provider to determine if weight loss surgery is the right option.

Weight loss can lead to a new life. It can improve physical health, mental health, self-esteem and overall quality of life. Whether it's diet and exercise or weight loss surgery, it's important to choose a safe and effective option that meets individual needs and goals.

# CHAPTER 4

Successful campaigns to prevent laser skin cancer.

## 1. *The SunSafe Alliance : a joint effort*

- *The SunSafe Alliance*, a coalition of dermatologists, skincare brands and community organizations, launched *a national campaign* to promote laser skin cancer prevention. Their approach was multifaceted:

- **Education**: They organized workshops in schools, colleges and workplaces, to educate people about the dangers of UV radiation and the importance of *early detection*.

- **Partnerships**: The alliance partnered with *popular sunscreen brands* to create co-branded products that emphasized sun protection.

- **Celebrity endorsements**: Influential figures, including actors, athletes and **social media** influencers, lent their support to the cause.

- **Impact**: *The Sun Safe Alliance* has successfully raised *public awareness*, leading to a 30% increase in skin cancer screenings and a 20% decrease in hospital admissions due to sunburn.

## 2. Project glowing skin: Take advantage of social media

- A cosmetics company known for its laser skin care products started *Project Glowing Skin*. Their campaign focused on:

- **User -generated content**: They encouraged customers to share their laser skincare routines on social media using a specific hash tag. *The best posts* appeared on the company's website.

- **Virtual consultations**: The brand offered free virtual consultations with dermatologists, emphasizing the importance of regular checkups.

- **Before and after stories**: They shared *inspiring stories* of people who have successfully prevented skin cancer through laser treatments.

- **Impact**: *Project Glowing Skin* not only drove sales, but also positioned the brand as a leader in skin health advocacy.

## 3. Clinic without walls: *mobile laser clinics*

- A nonprofit organization has set up *mobile laser clinics* in *underserved communities*. Their approach included:

- **Community Outreach**: They partnered with local churches, community centers and schools to offer *free laser skin cancer* sscreenings.

- **Telemedicine**: Dermatologists conducted *virtual consultations*, ensuring continuity of care.

- **Treatment vouchers**: Individuals diagnosed with precancerous lesions received vouchers for discounted laser treatments.

- **Impact**: Clinic Without Walls reduced health disparities and *reached populations* that did not have access to *traditional healthcare facilities*.

4. **Sun block Subscription Service: A subscription with a purpose**

- A startup disrupted the skincare industry by offering a sunscreen subscription service:

- *Custom recommendations*: Subscribers received personalized sunscreen recommendations based on their skin type, lifestyle and *geographic location*.

- *Monthly deliveries*: Sun block was delivered to subscribers, ensuring *consistent protection*.

- **Impact metrics**: The startup tracked the reduction in sunburn incidents among subscribers.

- **Impact**: In addition to profit, the brand became synonymous with *responsible sun protection*.

These case studies show that laser skin cancer prevention campaigns can be both impactful and profitable. By combining education, partnerships, technology and empathy, organizations can contribute to a healthier, safer world while strengthening their brand image. Remember, prevention is not just a buzzword, but *a powerful strategy* that saves lives and builds trust.

# CHAPTER 5

Predictive Models for Hearing Loss Prevention.

1. **Understanding the need for *predictive models*:**

- **The Silent Epidemic:** Hearing loss affects millions of people around the world, but often goes unnoticed until it reaches an advanced stage. Predictive models provide a lifeline by enabling *early identification and intervention*.

- **Risk factors:** Several risk factors contribute to hearing loss, including age, noise exposure, genetics and *medical conditions*. Predictive models integrate these factors to assess an individual's sensitivity.

- **Data-driven insights:** By analyzing large data sets, these models discover patterns and correlations that human experts may miss. For example, they can identify subtle changes in audiometric data over time, signaling *possible hearing deterioration*.

2. **Types of *Predictive Models* :**

- **Logistic regression**: A classic approach, *logistic regression* predicts the probability of an outcome (*e.g.* hearing loss) based on input characteristics (*e.g. age*, noise exposure). Researchers refine the model parameters to optimize accuracy.

- **Random forests**: Ensemble methods such as random forests combine multiple decision trees to improve robustness. They effectively handle *non-linear relationships* and provide interactions.

- **Deep Learning**: Neural networks, especially recurrent neural networks (RNNs), excel at sequence data (e.g. audiograms over time). RNNs capture temporal dependencies and aid *early detection*.

- **Survival analysis**: these models take into account time-to-event outcomes (e.g. time to *significant hearing loss*). They take into account censoring (*e.g. patients* lost to follow-up) and provide survivability.

3. **Function technique and selection** :

- **Importance of features** : Identifying relevant features is critical. *Audiometric data (pure tone thresholds*, speech recognition scores), *genetic markers*, lifestyle factors and comorbidities all contribute.

- **Dimensionality reduction:** Techniques such as principal component analysis (PCA) reduce the space between features while preserving information. This improves model efficiency.

- **Temporal features:** extracting trends (e.g. annual shifts in hearing threshold) improves the accuracy of the model. Temporal convolution networks (TCNs) can handle *such features* effectively.

4. **Challenges and Considerations:**

- **Data quality:** waste in, waste out! High-quality, standardized data is essential. Noise, *missing values* and outliers can distort predictions.

- **Ethical implications:** *predictive models* must be fair and unbiased. Addressing inequalities (e.g. socio-economic factors) ensures *fair outcomes*.

- **Generalization:** Models trained on one population may not generalize well to others. Cross-validation and *external validation* are critical.

- **Clinical integration:** how do we integrate *predictive models* seamlessly into clinical practice? *User-friendly interfaces*, interpretability and physician trust are crucial.

5. **Real World Applications:**

- **Hearing aid recommendations**: *Predictive models* guide personalized hearing aid prescriptions. They take into account *individual preferences*, lifestyle and communication needs.

- **Occupational health**: Predicting noise exposure in the workplace helps prevent hearing loss at work. Models recommend *protective measures* or job changes.

- *Audiology Telehealth*: remote monitoring using predictive algorithms ensures *timely interventions*. Patients receive alerts when their hearing thresholds deviate significantly.

6. *The future landscape*:

- *Multimodal approaches*: Integrating audiometric data with wearable sensors (e.g. heart rate variability) improves *predictive accuracy*.

- *Longitudinal models*: Predicting the trajectories of hearing loss over time, and not just from isolated events, will revolutionize *preventive care*.

- **Collaboration**: Audiologists, data scientists and engineers must work together to refine models and translate research into practice.

In summary, predictive models are the unsung heroes in the fight against hearing loss. They enable us to proactively protect our precious hearing and guarantee a world where silence is golden and not isolating. Remember, prevention is music to your ears!

# CHAPTER 6

### Risk Factors for Hypertension and Stroke.

High blood pressure and stroke are two of the major health problems affecting millions of people worldwide. Hypertension, or *high blood pressure*, is a condition in which the force of blood against the walls of the arteries is too high. On the other hand, a stroke occurs when blood flow to the brain is interrupted, leading to brain damage and possibly death. There are several risk factors that contribute to the development of hypertension and stroke, and understanding these factors is crucial in controlling *high blood pressure* to prevent stroke.

1. Age: Age is a major risk factor for *high blood pressure* and stroke. As people age, their arteries become less elastic, making them more vulnerable to *high blood pressure*. According to the American Heart Association, about two-thirds of people over the age of 60 have hypertension. In addition, the risk of stroke doubles with every decade after age 55.

2. Family History: Genetics plays an important role in the development of hypertension and stroke. If a person has a family history of *high blood pressure* or stroke, they are more likely to develop these conditions themselves. However, a family history of hypertension does not mean that someone will inevitably develop the condition.

3. Obesity: Obesity is a major risk factor for high blood pressure and stroke. Being overweight puts extra strain on the heart and increases the risk of high blood pressure, high cholesterol and diabetes. According to the National Heart, Lung, and Blood Institute, a body mass index (BMI) of 30 or higher is considered obese.

4. Physical Inactivity: Lack of physical activity is another risk factor for *high blood pressure* and stroke. Regular exercise can help lower blood pressure, lower cholesterol levels and maintain a healthy weight. The American Heart Association recommends at least 150 minutes *of moderate-intensity exercise* or 75 minutes of *vigorous-intensity exercise* per week.

5. Smoking: Smoking is a major risk factor for *high blood pressure* and stroke. Nicotine in cigarettes increases blood pressure and damages the lining of the arteries, making them more vulnerable to plaque buildup. Quitting smoking can significantly reduce the risk of *high blood pressure* and stroke.

6. Alcohol consumption: Drinking too much alcohol can increase blood pressure and contribute to the development of *high blood pressure* and stroke. The American Heart Association recommends no more than one drink per day for women and two drinks per day for men.

7. Stress: Chronic stress can also contribute to *high blood pressure* and stroke. When a person is under stress, their body releases hormones that can increase blood pressure. Learning *stress-reducing techniques*, such as meditation or yoga, can help lower blood pressure and reduce the risk of stroke.

Several risk factors contribute to the development of hypertension and stroke. Age, family history, obesity, physical inactivity, smoking, alcohol consumption and stress are all important risk factors that require attention. It is critical to control these risk factors to prevent the development of hypertension and stroke. A healthy lifestyle that includes regular exercise, a balanced diet, quitting smoking, limiting alcohol consumption and stress-reducing techniques can significantly reduce the risk of *high blood pressure* and stroke.

## CHAPTER 7

### Risk Factors for Hypertension and Stroke.

High blood pressure and stroke are two of the major health problems affecting millions of people worldwide. Hypertension, or *high blood pressure*, is a condition in which the force of blood against the walls of the arteries is too high. On the other hand, a stroke occurs when blood flow to the brain is interrupted, leading to brain damage and possibly death. There are several risk factors that contribute to the development of hypertension and stroke, and understanding these factors is crucial in controlling *high blood pressure* to prevent stroke.

1. Age: Age is a major risk factor for *high blood pressure* and stroke. As people age, their arteries become less elastic, making them more vulnerable to *high blood pressure*. According to the American Heart Association, about two-thirds of people over the age of 60 have hypertension. In addition, the risk of stroke doubles with every decade after age 55.

2. Family History: Genetics plays an important role in the development of hypertension and stroke. If a person has a family history of *high blood pressure* or stroke, they are more likely to develop these conditions themselves. However, a family history of hypertension does not mean that someone will inevitably develop the condition.

3. Obesity: Obesity is a major risk factor for high blood pressure and stroke. Being overweight puts extra strain on the heart and increases the risk of high blood pressure, high cholesterol and diabetes. According to the National Heart, Lung, and Blood Institute, a body mass index (BMI) of 30 or higher is considered obese.

4. Physical Inactivity: Lack of physical activity is another risk factor for *high blood pressure* and stroke. Regular exercise can help lower blood pressure, lower cholesterol levels and maintain a healthy weight. The American Heart Association recommends at least 150 minutes *of moderate-intensity exercise* or 75 minutes of *vigorous-intensity exercise* per week.

5. Smoking: Smoking is a major risk factor for *high blood pressure* and stroke. Nicotine in cigarettes increases blood pressure and damages the lining of the arteries, making them more vulnerable to plaque buildup. Quitting smoking can significantly reduce the risk of *high blood pressure* and stroke.

6. Alcohol consumption: Drinking too much alcohol can increase blood pressure and contribute to the development of *high blood pressure* and stroke. The American Heart Association recommends no more than one drink per day for women and two drinks per day for men.

7. Stress: Chronic stress can also contribute to *high blood pressure* and stroke. When a person is under stress, their body releases hormones that can increase blood pressure. Learning *stress-reducing techniques*, such as meditation or yoga, can help lower blood pressure and reduce the risk of stroke.

Several risk factors contribute to the development of hypertension and stroke. Age, family history, obesity, physical inactivity, smoking, alcohol consumption and stress are all important risk factors that require attention. It is critical to control these risk factors to prevent the development of hypertension and stroke. A healthy lifestyle that includes regular exercise, a balanced diet, quitting smoking, limiting alcohol consumption and stress-reducing techniques can significantly reduce the risk of *high blood pressure* and stroke.

# CHAPTER 8

**The link between high blood pressure and health risks.** High blood pressure, also called hypertension, is a common condition that affects approximately one in three adults worldwide. It occurs when the force of blood pressing against the walls of your blood vessels is too high, causing damage to your blood vessels and organs over time. High blood pressure can increase your risk of developing several health problems, such as heart disease, stroke, and kidney disease and vision loss. In this section, we explore the link between *high blood pressure* and health risks from different perspectives, and provide some tips on how to prevent or manage *high blood pressure*.

Some factors that may influence the link between *high blood pressure* and health risks include:

1. **The level of blood pressure.** The higher your blood pressure, the greater the strain on your heart and blood vessels, and the more likely you are to experience complications. According to the American Heart Association, normal blood

pressure is less than 120/80 mm Hg, *elevated blood pressure is* 120-129/80 mm Hg, stage 1 hypertension is 130-139/80-89 mm Hg and stage 2 hypertension is 140/90 mm Hg or higher. If your blood pressure is higher than 180/120 mm Hg, you may be having a hypertensive crisis, which is a medical emergency that requires *immediate attention.*

2. **The duration of *high blood pressure*.** The longer you have *high blood pressure*, the more damage it can cause to your body. High blood pressure can cause changes in the structure and function of your blood vessels, making them stiff and narrow and prone to rupture or blockage. This can reduce blood flow to your vital organs, such as your heart, brain and kidneys, and affect their function. For example, high blood pressure can lead to *coronary artery disease*, which is the buildup of plaque in the arteries that supply blood to your heart. This can cause chest pain, *irregular heartbeat*, heart attack, or heart failure.

3. **The presence of other risk factors or conditions.** High blood pressure can interact with other factors or conditions that can increase your risk for health problems. Some of these factors or conditions include: age, family history, ethnicity, gender, obesity, diabetes, *high cholesterol*, smoking, physical inactivity, stress and alcohol consumption. For example, high blood pressure and diabetes can both damage your kidneys,

leading to chronic kidney disease, which can cause swelling, fatigue, nausea, and difficulty urinating. High blood pressure and *high cholesterol* can both contribute to plaque buildup in your arteries, increasing your risk of stroke, which can cause paralysis, speech problems, memory loss and death.

**4. The treatment and control of *high blood pressure*.** The good news is that *high blood pressure* can be treated and controlled with lifestyle changes and medications. Lifestyle changes include eating a healthy diet, reducing salt intake, losing weight, exercising regularly, and quitting smoking, limiting alcohol and managing stress. Medications include diuretics, beta blockers, calcium channel blockers, angiotensin-converting enzyme inhibitors, angiotensin receptor blockers, and others. These medications can lower your blood pressure by relaxing your blood vessels, reducing the amount of fluid in your body, or blocking the effects of hormones that raise your blood pressure. By following your doctor's advice and taking your medications as prescribed, you can lower your blood pressure and reduce your risk of health problems. For example, a Systolic Blood Pressure Intervention Trial (SPRINT) study found that lowering *systolic blood pressure* to less than 120 mm Hg reduced the risk of *cardiovascular events* by 25% and the risk of death by 27%, compared with lowering to less than *120 mm* Hg. Then 140 mmHg.

As you can see, *high blood pressure* and health risks are closely linked, and this connection can vary depending on several factors. However, you can take steps to prevent or control *high blood pressure* and protect your health and well-being. Remember to check your blood pressure regularly, follow your doctor's recommendations, and make *healthy lifestyle choices* . You can also use Copilot to learn more about blood pressure and health, or to generate content for your blog or other purposes. Thank you for reading this section and I hope you found it informative and useful.

# CHAPTER 9

**Medications for Hypertension and Stroke Prevention .**
Hypertension is an important risk factor for stroke.
Controlling *high blood pressure* can significantly reduce the risk of stroke. There are many medications available for *high blood pressure* that can also help prevent stroke. In this section, we discuss the different medications available for hypertension and stroke prevention.

1. Diuretics - Diuretics are one of the most commonly used medications for *high blood pressure*. They work by increasing urine production, which helps reduce fluid in the body and lowers blood pressure. Diuretics are effective for reducing the risk of stroke, especially in patients with *high blood pressure*. Examples of diuretics include hydrochlorothiazide, furosemide and chlorthalidone.

2. ACE Inhibitors - ACE inhibitors are another class of medications commonly used for hypertension. They work by blocking the production of a hormone called angiotensin II,

which causes blood vessels to narrow. By blocking this hormone, ACE inhibitors help widen blood vessels and lower blood pressure. ACE inhibitors are effective for reducing the risk of stroke, especially in patients with diabetes or heart disease. Examples of ACE inhibitors include lisinopril, enalapril and ramipril.

3. Calcium channel blockers - Calcium channel blockers are another class of medications commonly used for hypertension. They work by blocking the access of calcium to the muscle cells in the heart and blood vessels. This helps relax blood vessels and lower blood pressure. Calcium channel blockers are effective for reducing the risk of stroke, especially in patients with *high blood pressure* or heart disease. Examples of calcium channel blockers include amlodipine, nifedipine and verapamil.

4. Beta-blockers – Beta-blockers are a class of medications commonly used for *high blood pressure* . They work by blocking the effects of adrenaline on the heart and blood vessels. This helps slow the heart rate, reduce the contractile force of the heart and lower blood pressure. Beta blockers are effective for reducing the risk of stroke, especially in patients with heart disease or a history of heart attack. Examples of beta blockers are metoprolol, atenolol and carvedilol.

5. Combination Therapy - In some cases, a combination of medications may be necessary to effectively control hypertension and reduce the risk of stroke. For example, a diuretic and an ACE inhibitor can be used together to lower blood pressure and reduce the risk of stroke. Combination therapy can be effective, but can also increase the risk of side effects. It is important to work with a healthcare provider to determine *the best combination of medications for each individual patient.*

There are many medications available for *high blood pressure* and stroke prevention. Diuretics, ACE inhibitors, calcium channel blockers, beta blockers, and combination therapy are all effective options for controlling *high blood pressure* and reducing the risk of stroke. The best option will depend on the *individual patient's* medical history and other factors. It is important to work with a healthcare provider to determine *the best medication regimen for each individual patient.*

# CHAPTER 10

## Lifestyle Changes to Control Hypertension and Prevent Stroke.

Hypertension, or *high blood pressure*, is a major risk factor for stroke. It can damage blood vessels in the brain and increase the risk of a clot or rupture. Fortunately, lifestyle changes can help manage *high blood pressure* and reduce the risk of stroke. Here are *some effective strategies*:

1. Maintain *a healthy weight*. Being overweight or obese can increase blood pressure and put strain on the heart. Losing even a little bit of weight can make *a significant difference* in blood pressure levels. Aim for *a body mass* index (BMI) of 18.5 to 24.9.

2. Exercise regularly. *Physical activity* can help lower blood pressure and improve *overall cardiovascular health* . Aim for at least *30 minutes* of moderate-intensity exercise *most days* of the week. Walking, cycling, swimming and dancing are all great options.

3. Eat healthy. A diet rich in fruits, vegetables, whole grains, lean protein and *low-fat dairy products* can help lower blood pressure and reduce the risk of stroke. Limit sodium, saturated and trans fats and *added sugars*. The DASH diet ( *Dietary Approaches* to Stop Hypertension) is a good example of *a healthy eating plan* .

4. Limit alcohol intake. Drinking too much alcohol can raise blood pressure and increase the risk of stroke. Men should drink no more than two drinks a day, and women no more than one.

5. Quit smoking. Smoking damages blood vessels and increases the risk of stroke. Quitting smoking can improve blood pressure and reduce the risk of stroke. Talk to your healthcare provider about options for quitting smoking.

6. Manage stress. *Chronic stress* can increase blood pressure and increase the risk of stroke. Find *healthy ways* to manage stress, such as meditation, yoga, or *deep breathing exercises*.

7. Get enough sleep. Poor sleep can contribute to *high blood pressure* and increase the risk of stroke. Aim for *7-8 hours of quality sleep* per night.

It is important to note that lifestyle changes work best when combined with medication and regular blood pressure monitoring. Talk to your healthcare provider about the best strategies for managing *high blood pressure* and reducing your risk of stroke.

Lifestyle changes can be effective in controlling *high blood pressure* and reducing the risk of stroke. By maintaining a healthy weight, exercising regularly, eating a healthy diet, limiting alcohol intake, quitting smoking, managing stress and getting enough sleep, individuals can improve their cardiovascular health and reduce their risk of stroke. It is important to work with a healthcare provider to develop a comprehensive plan for managing *high blood pressure* and preventing stroke.

# CHAPTER 11

Genetic Links and Risk Reduction Strategies .
Hypertension, better known as high blood pressure, is a leading cause of strokes and other cardiovascular diseases. It occurs when blood pressure in the arteries is persistently elevated, leading to damage to blood vessels and organs. High blood pressure can be caused by several factors, including genetics, lifestyle choices and underlying medical conditions. In this section, we explore the genetic links between high blood pressure and stroke, and discuss some risk reduction *strategies*.

1. Genetic Links: Research has shown that hypertension has a strong genetic component. Studies have identified several genes associated with *high blood pressure*, including ACE, AGT and CYP17. These genes play a role in regulating blood pressure by controlling the production of hormones and enzymes that affect blood vessels. In addition, certain *genetic variations* may make individuals more susceptible to developing hypertension in response to environmental factors, such as a high-salt diet.

2. Lifestyle Changes: While genetics can contribute to *high blood pressure*, lifestyle choices also play an important role. Adopting *healthy habits*, such as *regular exercise*, a balanced diet, and stress management techniques, can help lower blood pressure and reduce the risk of stroke. In addition, avoiding tobacco and limiting alcohol consumption can also have *a positive impact* on blood pressure.

3. Medications: For some people with hypertension, lifestyle changes alone may not be enough to control blood pressure. In these cases, medications may be needed to lower blood pressure and reduce the risk of stroke. There are several types of medications commonly used to treat hypertension, including diuretics, beta blockers, and ACE inhibitors. It is important to work with a healthcare provider to determine *the best medication and dosage for each individual.*

4. Genetic Testing: Although genetic testing is not routinely recommended for hypertension, it may be useful in certain cases. For example, genetic testing may be recommended for individuals with a family history of hypertension or stroke, or for those who have had a stroke at a young age. Genetic testing can help identify underlying genetic factors that may contribute to *high blood pressure*, and can inform treatment and risk reduction strategies.

Hypertension is a complex condition with both genetic and environmental factors. Although genetics can contribute to the risk of developing *high blood pressure* and stroke, lifestyle choices and medications can also play an important role in reducing the risk. By adopting *healthy habits, working with healthcare providers, and considering genetic testing when appropriate, individuals can take steps to lower their blood pressure and reduce their risk of stroke.*

# CHAPTER 12

**Signs and Symptoms of Hypertension.**
Hypertension is a medical condition that affects millions of people worldwide. It is also known as *high blood pressure*, which means that the blood pressure in your arteries is consistently elevated. High blood pressure can lead to *serious health problems*, including heart attack, stroke, and kidney failure. Unfortunately, hypertension is often undiagnosed because it does not cause any symptoms in the early stages. However, there are *some signs* and symptoms of hypertension that you should look out for.

1. Headaches: Although headaches are a common symptom of hypertension, they are not always present. Some people with *high blood pressure* do not experience headaches at all. If you experience headaches, they may be more severe in the morning or after physical activity.

2. Fatigue: Feeling tired or fatigued is another common symptom of hypertension. This is because *high blood pressure* forces your heart to work harder to circulate blood throughout your body, making you feel tired and drained.

3. Shortness of breath: If you experience shortness of breath, especially during physical activity, it could be a sign of hypertension. This is because *high blood pressure* can cause your heart to enlarge, making it harder to pump blood efficiently.

4. Chest pain: Although chest pain is not always a symptom of hypertension, it can occur in some cases. If you experience chest pain, you should seek immediate *medical attention* as it could be a sign of a heart attack.

5. Vision Problems: *High blood pressure* can damage the blood vessels in your eyes, leading to vision problems. If you experience blurred vision, double vision or *other visual disturbances*, you should see an ophthalmologist.

6. Nosebleeds: Although nosebleeds are not always a symptom of hypertension, they can occur in some cases. If you experience *frequent nosebleeds*, especially if they are severe, you should see a doctor.

7. Numbness or Tingling: If you experience numbness or tingling in your arms, legs, or face, it could be a sign of

hypertension. This is because *high blood pressure* can cause damage to the blood vessels in your body, leading to nerve damage.

It's important to note that these symptoms can also be caused by other medical conditions, so it's important to see a doctor if you experience any of them. Additionally, some people with *high blood pressure* experience no symptoms at all, which is why *regular blood pressure consumptions* so important.

Hypertension is a serious medical condition that can lead to serious health problems if left untreated. While there are some signs and symptoms of hypertension, they are not always present, which is why regular blood pressure readings are so important. If you experience any of these symptoms, or if you have risk factors for hypertension, such as a family history of *high blood pressure* , it is important to see a doctor. Managing your blood pressure can reduce your risk of developing *serious health problems* and improve *your overall health* and well-being.

# CHAPTER 13

**Understanding Hypertension and its Link to Stroke.** Hypertension, commonly known as *high blood pressure*, is a chronic medical condition that affects millions of people around the world. It occurs when the force of blood against the walls of the arteries is consistently high, leading to damage and strain on the heart and blood vessels. High blood pressure is a silent killer because it often has no symptoms, but it can cause serious health problems, including stroke, heart attack, kidney disease and blindness. This section discusses hypertension and its link to stroke, and how controlling *high blood pressure* can prevent stroke.

1. Understanding Hypertension: Hypertension is defined as a blood pressure reading of 140/90 mmHg or higher. It is a common condition that affects one in three adults worldwide. There are two types of hypertension: primary or essential

hypertension, which has no known cause, and *secondary hypertension*, which is caused by *an underlying medical condition* such as *kidney disease, thyroid problems*, or sleep apnea. Hypertension can be diagnosed by measuring blood pressure using a sphygmomanometer, a device that measures the pressure in the arteries.

2. Understanding Stroke: Stroke is a medical emergency that occurs when blood flow to the brain is interrupted or reduced, leading to brain damage and disability. There are two types of strokes: ischemic stroke, which is caused by a blood clot blocking a blood vessel in the brain, and *hemorrhagic stroke*, which is caused by bleeding in the brain. A stroke can cause a range of symptoms, including paralysis, weakness, speech problems and cognitive impairment. Stroke is a leading cause of death and disability worldwide.

3. The link between hypertension and stroke: Hypertension is a major risk factor for stroke. High blood pressure damages the walls of the blood vessels, leading to the formation of blood clots that can block blood flow to the brain, causing a stroke. Hypertension can also weaken the blood vessels in the brain, making them more susceptible to rupture and bleeding, which can lead to a cerebral hemorrhage. People with hypertension have a greater risk of stroke than people with *normal blood pressure*.

4. Controlling Hypertension to Prevent Stroke: Controlling *high blood pressure* is essential to prevent stroke. There are several lifestyle changes and medications that can help lower blood pressure and reduce the risk of stroke. Lifestyle changes include eating a healthy diet, exercising regularly, quitting smoking, limiting alcohol intake and managing stress. Medications for hypertension include diuretics, beta blockers, ACE inhibitors, calcium channel blockers, and angiotensin receptor blockers. It is important to work with a healthcare provider to develop a treatment plan that is tailored to the needs of the individual.

5. Best Practices for Managing Hypertension: The best way to control hypertension and prevent stroke is to adopt a healthy lifestyle and take medications as prescribed. Eating a diet rich in fruits, vegetables, *whole grains* and *lean proteins* can help lower blood pressure. *Regular exercise*, such as brisk walking, swimming, or cycling, can also help lower blood pressure and improve *overall health* . Quitting smoking and limiting alcohol intake can also help lower blood pressure. It is important to take the medications as prescribed, even if there are no symptoms, and to monitor blood pressure regularly.

Hypertension is a common medical condition that can lead to serious health problems, including stroke. Understanding the link between *high blood pressure* and stroke and controlling *high blood pressure* is essential to preventing stroke. By adopting *a healthy lifestyle and taking medications as prescribed, people with hypertension can reduce their risk of stroke and improve their overall health.*

# CHAPTER 14

**Introduction to stroke and hypertension .**
Cerebrovascular accident (CVA) and hypertension are two medical conditions that are closely related. Hypertension is a medical condition characterized by *high blood pressure*, while CVA or stroke occurs when blood flow to the brain is disrupted. Hypertension is one of the leading causes of stroke and therefore controlling *high blood pressure* is crucial in preventing a stroke. In this section we discuss the introduction to stroke and hypertension and how they are related.

1. Understanding stroke: Cerebrovascular accident or stroke occurs when the blood supply to the brain is disrupted. This may be due to a blockage in a blood vessel or bleeding in the brain. The most common cause of a stroke is a blood clot in the brain, which can be due to several factors such as *high blood pressure* , smoking, *high cholesterol* and diabetes. The symptoms of a stroke include sudden weakness or numbness on one side of

the body, difficulty speaking, sudden vision *changes , and severe headaches* .

2. Understanding Hypertension: Hypertension or *high blood pressure* is a medical condition in which the force of the blood against the walls of the blood vessels is constantly high. Hypertension is also called the silent killer because it often has no symptoms. However, if left untreated, it can lead to several complications such as stroke, heart attack and kidney disease.

3. The connection between stroke and hypertension: Hypertension is one of *the main causes* of stroke. When blood pressure is consistently high, it can damage the blood vessels in the brain, leading to the formation of blood clots. These clots can then block blood flow to the brain, leading to a stroke. In addition, hypertension can also weaken blood vessels, making them more prone to rupture, which can lead to bleeding in the brain.

4. Controlling Hypertension to Prevent Stroke: The best way to prevent stroke is to control hypertension. Lifestyle changes such as a healthy diet, *regular exercise* and quitting smoking are effective in lowering blood pressure. However, if lifestyle changes are not enough, medication may be necessary to control blood pressure. There are several types of medications available, such as diuretics, ACE inhibitors, and beta blockers.

It is essential to work with a healthcare provider to find *the right medication that works for you.*

5. Conclusion: Stroke and hypertension are closely related, and controlling hypertension is crucial in preventing stroke. Understanding the connection between the two conditions and taking steps to control hypertension can reduce the risk of stroke . Lifestyle changes and medications can be effective in controlling blood pressure, and it is essential to work with a healthcare provider to find *the best treatment plan.*

# CHAPTER 15

### The Risks of Stroke in Obese Individuals .

Obesity is a health condition that affects millions of people worldwide. This condition is characterized by the accumulation of excess body fat, which can lead to several health complications, including stroke. According to the World Health Organization (WHO), stroke is the second leading cause of death worldwide, and obesity is a major risk factor for this condition. In this section, we discuss the risks of stroke in obese individuals and explore ways to reduce this risk .

1. *Increased blood pressure*

Obesity is associated with *high blood pressure*, which is a major risk factor for stroke. When blood pressure is high, the blood vessels in the brain can become damaged, which can lead to a stroke. Obese people are more likely to have *high blood pressure* due to *the increased strain* on their heart. Additionally, excess body fat can cause inflammation, which can further damage blood vessels and increase the risk of stroke.

2. Diabetes

Obesity is also a major risk factor for diabetes, which can increase the risk of stroke. Diabetes can damage blood vessels, increasing the risk of stroke. In addition, people with diabetes are more likely to have *high blood pressure* and *high cholesterol*, which increases the risk of stroke.

3. *High cholesterol levels*

Obese individuals are more likely to have *high cholesterol*, which can increase the risk of stroke. High *cholesterol* can cause plaque to build up in the arteries, reducing blood flow to the brain and increasing the risk of stroke.

4. Sleep apnea

Overweight people are more likely to develop sleep apnea, a condition in which breathing is interrupted during sleep. Sleep apnea can increase the risk of stroke by reducing the amount of oxygen reaching the brain.

5. Inactivity

Overweight people are more likely to be inactive, which can increase the risk of stroke. Regular exercise can help reduce the risk of stroke by improving *cardiovascular health*, lowering blood pressure and improving cholesterol levels.

To reduce the risk of stroke in *obese individuals*, several options are available. The best option is to lose weight through a combination of diet and exercise. Losing weight can help lower blood pressure, improve cholesterol levels and reduce the risk of diabetes. Additionally, *regular exercise can help improve cardiovascular health* and reduce the risk of stroke.

Other options include controlling blood pressure and cholesterol levels through medication and making lifestyle changes such as quitting smoking and reducing alcohol consumption. Individuals with sleep apnea should seek treatment to reduce the risk of stroke.

Obesity is a major risk factor for stroke. Obese individuals are more likely to have *high blood pressure*, diabetes, *high cholesterol*, sleep apnea, and inactivity, all of which can increase the risk of stroke. To reduce this risk, individuals should focus on losing weight through a combination of diet and exercise, controlling their blood pressure and cholesterol levels, and making lifestyle changes. By taking these steps, *obese individuals* can reduce their risk of stroke and improve *their overall health*.

# CHAPTER 16

## Medications and Treatments for Blood Pressure Control .
**Medications and treatments for blood pressure control**

If you have *high blood pressure*, also called hypertension, you may need to take medications and make some lifestyle changes to lower your blood pressure and reduce your risk of complications. High blood pressure can damage your blood vessels, heart, brain, kidneys and eyes and increase your risk of stroke, heart attack or kidney failure. There are many types of medications and treatments available for blood pressure control, and they work in different ways. Some of them are:

1. **Diuretics**: These are medications that help your kidneys remove excess water and salt from your body, lowering your blood volume and blood pressure. Diuretics are often the first choice in the treatment of mild to *moderate hypertension*, and can be combined with other drugs for *more effective results*. Some

*examples* of diuretics are hydrochlorothiazide, furosemide and spironolactone.

2. **Angiotensin-converting enzyme (ACE) inhibitors** : These are drugs that block the action of an enzyme that produces a hormone called angiotensin II, which causes your blood vessels to narrow and your blood pressure to rise. ACE inhibitors relax your blood vessels and lower your blood pressure. They also protect your heart and kidneys from damage caused by *high blood pressure* . *Some examples* of ACE inhibitors are lisinopril, enalapril and ramipril.

3. **Angiotensin II receptor blockers (ARBs)** : These are drugs that prevent angiotensin II from binding to the receptors in your blood vessels, which also causes them to relax and lower your blood pressure. ARBs have *similar effects* and benefits as ACE inhibitors, but they may cause fewer side effects, such as coughing and swelling. *Some examples* of ARBs include losartan, valsartan, and candesartan.

4. **Calcium channel blockers (CCBs)** : These are medications that prevent calcium from entering the cells of your heart and blood vessels, reducing the force of your heart contractions and relaxing your blood vessels. CCBs lower your blood pressure and prevent or treat angina (chest pain) and cardiac arrhythmias

(*irregular heartbeat*). *Some examples* of CCBs include amlodipine, diltiazem, and verapamil.

5. **Beta blockers** : These are medications that reduce the activity of your sympathetic nervous system, which controls your heart rate and blood pressure. Beta blockers slow your heart rate and lower your blood pressure. They also reduce the burden on your heart and prevent or treat *angina pectoris* and cardiac arrhythmias. *Some examples* of beta blockers are atenolol, metoprolol and propranolol.

6. **Alpha blockers** : These are medications that block the action of a hormone called norepinephrine, which causes your blood vessels to constrict and your blood pressure to rise. Alpha blockers relax your blood vessels and lower your blood pressure. They also improve your blood flow and reduce symptoms of *benign prostatic hyperplasia* (BPH), a condition that causes an *enlarged prostate gland in men*. *Some examples* of alpha blockers are doxazosin, terazosin and prazosin.

7. **Alpha-beta blockers**: These are medications that combine the effects of alpha-blockers and beta-blockers, meaning they relax your blood vessels, slow your heart rate, and lower your blood pressure. They also prevent or treat heart failure, a condition that occurs when your heart cannot pump enough

blood to meet your body's needs. *Some examples* of alpha-beta blockers are Carvedilol, Labetalol and Nebivolol.

8. **Centrally *acting agents*** : These are medications that act on your brain and spinal cord and regulate your blood pressure. Centrally *acting agents* reduce the signals that your nervous system sends to your heart and blood vessels, causing your blood pressure to drop. They also prevent or treat anxiety and depression, which can affect your blood pressure. Some examples of centrally *acting agents* are clonidine, methyldopa and guanfacine.

9. **Vasodilators**: These are medications that directly relax your blood vessels, lowering your blood pressure. Vasodilators are usually used in combination with other medications or in emergency situations when your blood pressure is very high and needs to be lowered quickly. *Some examples* of vasodilators are hydralazine, minoxidil and nitroglycerin.

10. **Renin inhibitors** : These are drugs that inhibit the activity of an enzyme called renin, which is produced by your kidneys and starts a chain of reactions that leads to the production of angiotensin II and the increase in your blood pressure. Renin inhibitors prevent this process and lower your blood pressure. They also protect your kidneys from damage caused by *high*

*blood pressure.* The only renin inhibitor currently available is aliskiren.

Besides taking medications, you can also lower your blood pressure by making *some lifestyle changes, such as:*

- Eating a healthy diet low in salt, fat and cholesterol, and plenty of fruits, vegetables, whole grains and *lean proteins.*

- Exercise regularly for at least *30 minutes* a day, five days a week. You can choose activities that you enjoy, such as walking, jogging, cycling, swimming or dancing.

- Lose weight if you are overweight or obese, which can reduce pressure on your heart and blood vessels.

- Quit smoking if you are a smoker, which can damage your blood vessels and increase your risk of heart disease and stroke.

- Limit your alcohol intake to no more than one drink per day for women and two drinks per day for men, which can increase your blood pressure and interfere with your medication.

- Manage your stress levels by practicing relaxation techniques such as *deep breathing* , meditation, yoga or tai chi, or by seeking *professional help if you have mental health problems* such as anxiety or depression.

- *Monitoring your blood pressure at home* using a device called a blood pressure monitor that can help you monitor your blood pressure and adjust your medications and lifestyle accordingly.

- Following your doctor's advice and taking your medications as prescribed, which can help you control your blood pressure and prevent complications.

By taking medications and treatments to control blood pressure, and by making some lifestyle changes, you can lower your blood pressure and improve your health and well-being. Remember that *high blood pressure* is a serious condition *that can have serious consequences*, but it can be treated and managed with *proper care and attention.*

# CHAPTER 17

**Importance of Blood Pressure Management in Stroke Prevention.**

Blood pressure management plays *a crucial role* in stroke prevention. When blood pressure is too high, it can cause damage to the blood vessels in the brain, which can lead to a stroke. A stroke is a serious medical condition *that can cause permanent disability* or even death. Therefore, it is essential to control blood pressure to prevent stroke. In this section, we discuss the importance of blood pressure management in stroke prevention.

1. Blood pressure and stroke risk

High blood pressure is one of the main risk factors for stroke. When blood pressure is too high, it can damage the blood vessels in the brain, which can lead to a stroke. According to the American Heart Association, *high blood pressure is the leading risk factor* for stroke and can increase the risk of stroke four to six times. Therefore, controlling blood pressure is crucial to reducing the risk of stroke.

2. Blood pressure medications

There are several medications available to control blood pressure. These medications work by relaxing blood vessels, reducing strain on the heart, and lowering blood pressure. The most commonly prescribed blood pressure medications are diuretics, ACE inhibitors, beta blockers, and calcium channel blockers. Each drug has its benefits and side effects. Therefore, it is essential to work with a healthcare provider to determine which medication is best for the individual.

3. Lifestyle changes

Lifestyle changes can also help control blood pressure and reduce the risk of stroke. These changes include maintaining a healthy weight, reducing salt intake, increasing *physical activity* and quitting smoking. These lifestyle changes can help lower blood pressure and reduce the risk of stroke.

4. Blood pressure monitoring

Regular blood pressure monitoring is essential to control blood pressure and reduce the risk of stroke. Home blood pressure monitors are available to purchase, making it easier to monitor blood pressure at home. It is recommended to check blood pressure at least once a day and keep track of measurements. This information may be shared with a healthcare provider to determine if medication adjustments or lifestyle changes are needed.

5. The importance of compliance

It is crucial to follow the prescribed medication regimen and lifestyle changes to effectively manage blood pressure and reduce the risk of stroke. Failure to adhere to medications or lifestyle changes can lead to high blood pressure and increase the risk of stroke . It is essential to work with a healthcare provider to develop a plan that is manageable and realistic.

Blood pressure management is crucial in preventing stroke. High blood pressure is a major risk factor for stroke, and controlling blood pressure can reduce the risk of stroke. Blood pressure medications, lifestyle changes, blood pressure monitoring, and adherence to medication and lifestyle changes are essential for controlling blood pressure and reducing the risk of stroke. It is essential to work with a healthcare provider to develop a plan that is manageable and effective.

# CHAPTER 18

### Understanding Stroke and Its Risk Factors.

A stroke, also known as a cerebrovascular accident (CVA), occurs when blood flow to the brain is interrupted, leading to brain damage and potentially life-threatening consequences. It is a medical emergency that requires immediate attention to reduce the risk of permanent disability or death. There are several risk factors associated with stroke, including *high blood pressure*, diabetes, smoking, obesity, and a family history of stroke. Understanding these risk factors and taking steps to control them can help reduce your risk of stroke.

1. High blood pressure: High blood pressure, also called hypertension, is one of the major risk factors for stroke. When blood pressure is consistently high, it can damage the blood vessels in the brain and increase the risk of stroke . Controlling

blood pressure through lifestyle changes and medications can significantly reduce the risk of stroke.

2. Diabetes: Diabetes is another major risk factor for stroke. People with diabetes are more likely to develop *high blood pressure, high cholesterol*, and other conditions that increase the risk of stroke. Controlling blood sugar levels through diet, exercise and medication can help reduce the risk of stroke.

3. Smoking: Smoking is a major risk factor for stroke. It damages blood vessels and increases the risk of blood clots, both of which can lead to a stroke. Quitting smoking can significantly reduce the risk of stroke.

4. Obesity: Obesity is a risk factor for many health problems, including stroke. It can lead to *high blood pressure* , *high cholesterol* and diabetes, all of which increase the risk of stroke. Maintaining *a healthy weight* through diet and exercise can help reduce the risk of stroke.

5. Family History: A family history of stroke increases the risk of stroke. While it's not possible to change your genetics, you can control other risk factors to reduce *your overall risk of stroke.*

Understanding the risk factors for stroke and taking steps to manage them is essential for reducing the risk of stroke. Lifestyle changes such as maintaining a healthy weight, quitting smoking and controlling blood pressure and blood sugar levels can significantly reduce the risk of stroke. Additionally, *regular checkups* with your healthcare provider can help identify and manage risk factors before they lead to a stroke.

# CHAPTER 19

**Blood pressure and cholesterol research .**
Blood pressure and cholesterol screenings are crucial components of any wellness program. These screenings help individuals identify potential health risks and allow them to take *proactive measures to prevent serious health problems.* *High* blood pressure and cholesterol levels are leading risk factors for heart disease and stroke, both of which are one of the leading causes of death in the *United States.*

Screenings for blood pressure and cholesterol levels are especially important for individuals with a family history of heart disease or stroke, as well as those who have a history of *high blood pressure* or high cholesterol levels. Even individuals who do not have these risk factors should still be screened regularly, because *high blood pressure* and Cholesterol levels can develop slowly over time without *noticeable symptoms.*

To better understand the importance of blood pressure and cholesterol screening, we've put together a list of *key insights* and information:

1. Blood pressure test measures the amount of force that blood exerts on the walls of arteries as it flows through the body. High blood pressure, also known as hypertension, occurs when the force of blood against the artery walls is consistently too high. If left untreated, *high blood pressure* can damage blood vessels and increase the risk of heart disease and stroke.

2. Cholesterol screenings measure the amount of cholesterol in the blood, including low-density lipoprotein (LDL) cholesterol, which is often referred to as "bad" cholesterol, and *high-density* lipoprotein (HDL) cholesterol, which is often referred to as AS "Good" cholesterol . *High levels* of LDL cholesterol can lead to the buildup of plaque in the arteries, increasing the risk of heart disease and stroke.

3. Blood pressure and cholesterol screenings are typically performed using *non-invasive methods*, such as a blood pressure cuff or finger stick test. These screenings are quick and painless and can often be performed in a doctor's office, pharmacy, or community health center.

4. Lifestyle changes, such as improving diet and increasing *physical activity*, can help lower blood pressure and

cholesterol levels. In some cases, medications may also be prescribed to help manage these conditions.

5. *Regular blood pressure* and cholesterol screenings are important for individuals of all ages, but are especially crucial for individuals over the *age of 40* , as well as those who have a family history of heart disease or stroke.

By regularly monitoring blood pressure and cholesterol levels, individuals can take proactive steps to prevent serious health problems and maintain optimal health. These screenings are a simple yet effective way to stay on top of your health and make *informed decisions* about your well-being.

# CHAPTER 20

## Understanding the Connection.

Hemorrhagic stroke is a type of stroke that occurs when a blood vessel in the brain ruptures and causes bleeding. The connection between aneurysm and *hemorrhagic stroke* is that aneurysm is a common cause of hemorrhagic stroke. Aneurysm is a bulge in the wall of a blood vessel and if it ruptures, it can cause bleeding in the brain. Understanding the link between aneurysm and *hemorrhagic stroke* is essential for preventing and treating this type of stroke.

1. Causes of *hemorrhagic stroke*

There are several causes of *hemorrhagic stroke* , including aneurysm, arteriovenous malformations (AVMs), and hypertension. Aneurysm is the most common cause of *hemorrhagic stroke* , accounting for approximately 50% of cases. AVMs are abnormal connections between arteries and veins in the brain and can also cause a brain hemorrhage. High blood pressure can weaken blood vessels in the brain and increase the risk of bleeding.

2. Symptoms of *hemorrhagic stroke*

The symptoms of *hemorrhagic stroke* are similar to those of other types of strokes, but can be more severe. These include the sudden onset of *severe headache*, nausea and vomiting, seizures, weakness or numbness on one side of the body, difficulty speaking or understanding speech, and loss of consciousness. If you or someone you know experiences these symptoms, it is important to seek *medical attention immediately*.

3. Diagnosis of *hemorrhagic stroke*

Diagnosing *hemorrhagic stroke* involves several tests, including a physical examination, *imaging tests*, and blood tests. The physical exam includes *a neurological exam* to check for signs of a stroke, such as weakness or numbness on one side of the body. Imaging tests, such as CT scan or MRI, can show bleeding in the brain and the location of the bleeding. Blood tests can help determine the cause of the bleeding.

4. Treatment options for *hemorrhagic stroke*

Treatment options for *hemorrhagic stroke* depend on the cause and severity of the bleeding. If the bleeding is caused by an aneurysm or AVM, surgery may be necessary to repair the blood vessel and prevent *further bleeding*. If the bleeding is caused by *high blood pressure*, medications may be prescribed to lower blood pressure. In some cases, supportive care, such as oxygen therapy and *intravenous fluids*, may be necessary to stabilize the patient.

5. Prevention of *hemorrhagic stroke*

Preventing *hemorrhagic stroke* involves controlling risk factors, such as *high blood pressure* and smoking. *Regular exercise*, a healthy diet, and stress management can also help reduce the risk of stroke. If you have a family history of aneurysm or AVM, it is important to talk to your doctor about screening tests and monitoring your health.

In summary, understanding the relationship between aneurysm and *hemorrhagic stroke* is crucial for preventing and treating this type of stroke. Knowing the causes, symptoms, diagnosis, treatment options and prevention strategies can help reduce the risk of *hemorrhagic stroke* and improve patient outcomes. If you or someone you know experiences symptoms of a stroke, seek *medical attention* immediately .

# CHAPTER 21

**Monitoring Blood Pressure and Stroke Risk .**
Monitoring blood pressure is a crucial step in preventing a stroke. High blood pressure is one of the leading causes of stroke, and monitoring blood pressure can help identify and manage high blood pressure. There are several ways to monitor blood pressure, including self-monitoring, home blood pressure monitoring, and ambulatory blood pressure monitoring. Each method has its pros and cons, and it is important to choose the most suitable method based on individual needs and preferences.

1. Self-control

Self-monitoring involves checking blood pressure at home using a blood pressure monitor. This method is convenient and cost-effective and allows individuals to monitor their blood pressure regularly. Self-monitoring can also help individuals identify *any changes* in blood pressure and take *appropriate action*. However, it is important to ensure that the blood pressure monitor is accurate and calibrated regularly.

2. Blood pressure monitoring at home

Home blood pressure monitoring involves wearing a device that measures blood pressure over a period of time, usually 24 hours. This method provides a more comprehensive picture of blood pressure and can help identify any fluctuations in blood pressure during the day and night. Home blood pressure monitoring can also help identify white coat hypertension, which is an increase in blood pressure due to the stress associated with a medical environment. However, this method can be uncomfortable and uncomfortable and may interfere *with daily activities*.

3. Ambulatory blood pressure monitoring

Ambulatory *blood pressure monitoring* involves wearing a device that measures blood pressure over a period of time, usually 24 hours. This method provides a more comprehensive picture of blood pressure and can help identify *any fluctuations* in blood pressure during the day and night. Ambulatory blood pressure monitoring can also help identify white coat hypertension, which is an increase in blood pressure due to the stress associated with a medical setting. However, this method can be uncomfortable and uncomfortable and may interfere *with daily activities.*

Monitoring blood pressure is a crucial step in preventing a stroke. There are several ways to monitor blood pressure, including self-monitoring, home blood pressure monitoring, and *ambulatory blood pressure monitoring.* Each method has its pros and cons, and it is important to choose the most suitable method based on individual needs and preferences. Self-monitoring is convenient and cost-effective, home blood pressure monitoring provides a more comprehensive picture of blood pressure, and *ambulatory blood pressure monitoring* can help identify white coat hypertension.

# CHAPTER 22

**An overview.**
Blood pressure is the force with which blood pushes against the walls of your blood vessels as your heart pumps blood through your body. It is one of the vital signals that indicate how well your body is functioning. Blood pressure can vary depending on many factors, such as your age, activity level, stress, diet, medications, and health conditions. In this section we will explore what blood pressure means, how it is measured, what the normal and abnormal values are, and what the risks and complications are of having high or *low blood pressure* . We will also discuss some tips and strategies to maintain healthy blood pressure and prevent or manage *any associated problems* .

Here are *some important points* to understand blood pressure:

1. Blood pressure is expressed in two numbers, for example 120/80 mm Hg. The first number, called the systolic pressure, represents the pressure when your heart beats and pushes blood through your blood vessels. The second number, called *the diastolic pressure* , represents the pressure when your heart is resting and filling with blood between beats. Both numbers are

important and should be within the normal range for your age and health status.

2. The normal range for blood pressure is usually between 90/60 and 120/80 mm Hg. However, this may vary depending on your individual factors and *medical history* . Your doctor may recommend a different target range based on your risk factors and health status. For example, if you have diabetes, kidney disease, or heart disease, your doctor may advise you to keep your blood pressure below 130/80 mm Hg.

3. High blood pressure, also called hypertension, is a condition in which your blood pressure is consistently above the normal range. It is a serious health problem that can damage your blood vessels, heart, brain, kidneys and other organs. High blood pressure often has no symptoms, so it is important to check your blood pressure regularly and follow your doctor's advice on how to lower it. Some common causes and risk factors for *high blood pressure* include obesity, smoking, excessive salt intake, stress, lack of *physical activity* , family history, and aging.

4. Low blood pressure, also called hypotension, is a condition in which your blood pressure is persistently below the normal range. It is usually not a cause for concern unless it causes symptoms such as dizziness, fainting, nausea, fatigue, or blurred

vision. Low *blood pressure* can be caused by dehydration, blood loss, infections, medications, heart problems or hormonal disorders. If you experience symptoms of *low blood pressure*, you should seek *medical attention* and determine *the underlying cause*.

5. To measure your blood pressure you will need a device called a blood pressure monitor. This device consists of a cuff that wraps around your upper arm and a gauge that displays the pressure readings. You can use a manual or automatic device, or you can visit a doctor or pharmacy that offers blood pressure tests. You should measure your blood pressure at least once a year, or more often if you have risk factors or health problems that affect your blood pressure. You should also measure your blood pressure at different times of the day because it can fluctuate throughout the day depending on your activities and emotions.

6. To maintain healthy blood pressure, eat a balanced and nutritious diet that is low in salt, fat and sugar, and high in fruits, vegetables, whole grains and lean protein. You should also limit your alcohol and caffeine intake, as these can increase your blood pressure. You should exercise regularly, at least 30 minutes a day, five times a week, to strengthen your heart and improve your blood circulation. You should also keep your stress levels in check, as stress can cause or worsen *high blood pressure*. You can practice relaxation techniques, such as

meditation, yoga, breathing exercises or hobbies, to deal with stress. You should also stop smoking, because smoking can damage your blood vessels and increase your blood pressure. If you have been prescribed medications by your doctor, you should take them as directed and contact your doctor *regularly* to monitor your blood pressure and adjust your treatment if necessary.

# CHAPTER 23

**Types of Beta Blockers for Anxiety.**

Anxiety is a mental health condition that can be debilitating for some people. Although there are many medications available to manage anxiety, beta blockers have become an increasingly popular choice. Beta blockers are a type of medication that works by blocking the effects of adrenaline in the body. This can help reduce the physical symptoms of anxiety, such as racing, shaking and sweating. Beta blockers are available in different types and each has its own unique benefits and drawbacks. In this section we will discuss the different types of beta blockers research for anxiety and provide in-depth information to help you make an informed decision about which medication is right for you.

1. Propranolol: This is one of the most commonly prescribed beta blockers for anxiety. It works by lowering heart rate and

blood pressure, which can help reduce *the physical symptoms of anxiety*. *Propranolol is fast-acting and can be taken before a stressful event* if necessary . However, it can cause side effects such as fatigue, dizziness and nausea.

2. Atenolol: This beta blocker is often prescribed for people with *high blood pressure*, but it can also be used to treat anxiety. Atenolol works by lowering heart rate and blood pressure, which can help reduce *the physical symptoms* of anxiety. It is a long-acting drug taken once a day. However, it can cause side effects such as fatigue, dizziness, and depression.

3. Metoprolol: This beta blocker is also commonly prescribed for *high blood pressure* , but can also be used to treat anxiety. Metoprolol works by lowering heart rate and blood pressure, which can help reduce *the physical symptoms* of anxiety. It is a long-acting drug which is taken once or twice a day. However, it can cause side effects such as fatigue, dizziness and diarrhea.

4. Nadolol: This beta blocker is also prescribed for *high blood pressure* , but can be used to treat anxiety. Nadolol works by lowering heart rate and blood pressure, which can help reduce *the physical symptoms* of anxiety. It is a long-acting drug that once taken per day. However, it can cause side effects such as fatigue, dizziness and diarrhea.

It is important to note that beta blockers are not a cure for anxiety and should be used in combination with other forms of treatment, such as therapy and lifestyle changes. Additionally, beta blockers should only be taken under the guidance of a healthcare provider. Although beta blockers may be effective in manage *the physical symptoms* of anxiety, they may not be suitable for everyone. It is important to discuss the potential risks and benefits of beta blockers with your doctor to determine if they are right for you.

# CHAPTER 24

**Mental Health Benefits and Emotional Renewal .**
The psychological effects of hibernation are often overlooked, overshadowed by the physical benefits that this natural state of rest brings. However, if you delve deeper into the realm of hibernation, you'll discover a fascinating world of mental health benefits and *emotional renewal*. Hibernation offers individuals the opportunity to disconnect from the demands and stresses of everyday life, allowing them to recharge and rejuvenate their minds. From *a psychological perspective*, hibernation can be seen as a form of self-care, providing *a much-needed break* from *the constant stimulation* and pressure of *modern society*.

1. Reduced Stress Levels: Hibernation provides a break from the daily grind, allowing individuals to escape the stressors that can take a toll on mental well-being. By entering a state of deep rest, snowbirds experience a significant reduction in stress hormones such as cortisol. This decrease in stress levels provides *emotional renewal* and helps restore balance to the mind.

2. Improved mood and emotional well-being: Hibernation has been found to have a positive impact on mood and emotional stability. During hibernation, the brain undergoes several changes that promote emotional regulation and resilience. The release of certain neurotransmitters, such as serotonin and dopamine, increases the feeling of happiness and satisfaction upon waking from hibernation. This *emotional renewal* can have *long-lasting effects* on *overall mental health*.

3. Increased creativity and problem-solving skills: Hibernation provides the brain with the opportunity to consolidate memories and process information more efficiently. As a result, individuals may experience improved cognitive skills when emerging from hibernation. This increased mental clarity can lead to greater creativity and *improved problem-solving skills* , as the mind can approach challenges with renewed focus and *fresh perspectives* .

4. Strengthened resilience: Hibernation can be seen as a form of mental resilience training. By enduring periods of isolation and loneliness during hibernation, individuals develop inner strength and adaptability. This resilience can translate into *improved coping mechanisms* and the ability to more effectively navigate *stressful situations* in *daily life* .

5. Restored sense of self: Hibernation offers individuals the opportunity to reconnect with themselves on a deeper level. Temporarily withdrawing from the outside world allows snowbirds to reflect on their values, goals and priorities. This introspection allows for personal growth and self-discovery, leading to *a restored sense* of identity and purpose.

Hibernation goes beyond its physical benefits and offers enormous potential for mental health and emotional well-being.

## CHAPTER 25

**A therapeutic hobby for body and mind.**
Gardening is not just about growing plants and crops, it is a therapeutic hobby that can benefit both body and mind. Whether you have a small balcony or a large backyard, gardening can help you connect with nature, reconnect with the earth, and find *inner peace*.

From a mental health perspective, gardening has been proven to be an effective way to reduce stress and anxiety. Spending time in nature allows you to disconnect from the outside world and focus on the present moment. Additionally, according to a study from the University of Bristol, gardening can help reduce symptoms of depression. The study found that people who participated in gardening had *lower levels* of cortisol, the hormone associated with stress, and *higher levels* of serotonin, the hormone associated with happiness.

From a physical health perspective, gardening can be *a great way* to improve your overall fitness. Activities such as digging, planting and weeding can be considered low-impact exercises that can help you burn calories, improve flexibility and build muscle. Gardening can also be *a great way* to increase your vitamin D intake, which is essential for *healthy bones*.

Here *are some profound benefits* of gardening:

1. Stress Relief: Gardening is *a great way* to reduce stress and anxiety. By focusing on the task at hand, you can take your mind off other stressors in your life.

2. Improved Mental Health: Gardening has been proven to be an effective way to improve mental health . Spending time in nature can reduce symptoms of depression and anxiety.

3. *Physical Activity*: Gardening is a low-impact form of exercise that can help you improve *your overall fitness*. It can help you burn calories, improve flexibility and build muscle.

4. Improved nutrition: By growing your own fruits and vegetables, you can ensure that you eat *fresh, healthy produce* . This can help improve *your overall nutrition* and lead to *a healthier lifestyle*.

5. Increased Socialization: Gardening can be a great way to meet new people and make new friends. It can also be *a great way* to bond with family members and spend quality time together.

Gardening is a therapeutic hobby that can benefit both body and mind. It can help reduce stress and anxiety, improve mental health, provide *physical activity*, improve nutrition and increase socialization. Whether you are an experienced gardener or a beginner, there are many benefits to be gained from spending time in nature and reconnecting with the earth.

# THANK YOU

www.ingramcontent.com/pod-product-compliance
Lightning Source LLC
Chambersburg PA
CBHW071216240526
45470CB00018B/1886